CONTENTS

The Toxin Takedown 1

Introduction 3

Chapter 1: What is Detoxification? 9

Chapter 2: The Modern Toxic Landscape 14

Chapter 3: How Toxins Affect Your Body 18

Chapter 4: Your Body's Natural Detoxification Systems ... 24

Chapter 5: Detox for Teenagers: Building Healthy Habits ... 29

Chapter 6: Detox for Children: Protecting Their Growing Bodies ... 31

Chapter 7: Detox for Adults: Addressing Specific Concerns ... 34

Chapter 8: Detox for the Elderly: Maintaining Vitality ... 37

Chapter 9: Detox Diets: The Foundation of Detoxification ... 40

Chapter 10: Supplements and Herbs for Detoxification ... 44

Chapter 11: Lifestyle Practices for Detoxification ... 48

Chapter 12: Detoxification for Specific Conditions ... 52

Chapter 13: Creating a Toxin-Free Home Environment ... 60

Chapter 14: Choosing Safe and Effective Detox Products ... 65

Chapter 15: Building a Support System for Your Detox Journey ... 70

Appendix 74

THE TOXIN TAKEDOWN

A Practical Guide to Eliminating Toxins To Unleash Your Body's Natural Healing Powers

Gertrude Swanson

No part of this book may be reproduced or transmitted in any form whatsoever, electronic, or mechanical, including photocopying, recording, or by any informational storage or retrieval system without express permission from the author.

Copyright © 2024 JNR Publishing
All rights reserved

INTRODUCTION

The Importance of Detoxification in the Modern World

In today's fast-paced, technology-driven world, we are faced with an unprecedented level of exposure to toxins. This toxic landscape poses a unique challenge for individuals seeking to maintain optimal health and well-being.

The air we breathe is polluted with a myriad of harmful substances, including particulate matter, ozone, and toxic chemicals. These pollutants can irritate the lungs, cause respiratory problems, and increase the risk of cardiovascular disease and cancer.

The food we eat is often laden with pesticides, herbicides, and other chemicals that can disrupt our endocrine system, damage our organs, and contribute to chronic diseases such as obesity, diabetes, and cancer.

Even the water we drink may contain contaminants such as lead, mercury, and bacteria, which can cause a range of health problems, including gastrointestinal issues, neurological damage, and kidney disease.

In addition to environmental toxins, we are also exposed to a variety of toxins in our homes and workplaces. These can include cleaning products, personal care products, and building materials that release harmful chemicals into the air.

The cumulative effect of these toxins can take a significant toll on our health. They can contribute to fatigue, headaches, skin problems, digestive issues, and a weakened immune system. In some cases, exposure to toxins can lead to more serious health problems, such as cancer, reproductive disorders, and autoimmune diseases.

Individuals who are concerned about their exposure to toxins can take steps to reduce their risk. These steps include:

- Eating a healthy diet that is rich in fruits, vegetables, and whole grains.
- Choosing organic foods whenever possible.
- Filtering tap water or drinking bottled water.
- Using natural cleaning products and personal care products.
- Avoiding exposure to secondhand smoke.
- Spending time in nature.

By taking these steps, we can reduce our exposure to toxins and improve our overall health and well-being.

The Rising Toxic Burden: A 21st-Century Reality

One of the most pressing challenges of the 21st century is environmental pollution, a result of the exponential increase in synthetic chemicals used in industrial processes, agriculture, cosmetics, and many other everyday products. These chemicals have permeated our environment, contaminating our air, water, and soil.

Unfortunately, we are exposed to a greater variety and quantity of toxins than ever before. This constant exposure to pollutants can have a profound impact on our health. Research has linked exposure to environmental toxins with various health concerns, including respiratory problems, skin conditions, reproductive issues, and even cancer.

Understanding the impact of these substances on our health is paramount. It is essential to conduct comprehensive scientific studies to assess the toxicity levels of different chemicals and determine their potential effects on human health. Furthermore, raising awareness about the hazards of environmental toxins and promoting sustainable practices is crucial.

To mitigate the effects of environmental pollution, several proactive steps can be taken. One effective strategy is reducing our reliance on synthetic chemicals in agriculture and shifting towards more eco-friendly farming methods. Investing in renewable energy sources and implementing strict environmental regulations are also necessary measures to curb pollution.

On an individual level, we can make conscious choices to minimize our exposure to toxins. Simple actions such as avoiding the use of harsh chemicals in household cleaning products, choosing organic produce whenever possible, and opting for natural personal care products can make a significant difference.

Additionally, promoting a healthy lifestyle that includes a balanced diet rich in antioxidants, regular exercise, and adequate sleep can help strengthen our immune system and enhance our ability to combat the effects of environmental pollutants.

By taking a proactive approach, we can reduce our exposure to environmental toxins, safeguard our health, and ensure a sustainable future for generations to come. The 21st century presents unique challenges, but it also offers an opportunity to create a healthier and more sustainable world for ourselves and future generations.

Understanding the Impact of Toxins on Health

Toxins can have a profound impact on our physical and mental well-being. Chronic exposure to toxins has been linked to various health conditions, including digestive disorders, hormonal imbalances, cognitive decline, and even cancer. By understanding the mechanisms through which toxins affect our bodies, we can develop effective strategies to support our natural detoxification processes and promote optimal health.

Empowering Yourself Through Knowledge and Action

The path to a healthier, toxin-free life begins with education and empowerment. By arming yourself with the knowledge and tools necessary to navigate the modern toxic landscape, you can take control of your health and make informed decisions about your lifestyle choices. This book aims to provide you with a comprehensive understanding of detoxification and equip you with practical strategies to support your body's natural cleansing mechanisms.

How This Book Can Help You

"Detox Diets for the Modern Age" is designed to be your go-to resource for understanding and implementing effective detoxification strategies. Throughout the book, you will learn about:

- The science behind detoxification and how your body eliminates toxins
- The various sources of toxins in our modern environment and their impact on health
- Age-specific detoxification considerations for children, teenagers, adults, and seniors
- The principles and types of detox diets, along with meal planning and recipes
- Supplements, herbs, and lifestyle practices that support detoxification
- Strategies for creating a toxin-free home environment and choosing safe detox products
- Building a support system to help you stay motivated and overcome challenges

A Holistic Approach to Detoxification

In the realm of wellness, the concept of detoxification extends beyond mere physical cleansing. This book embraces a holistic perspective, acknowledging that true health and well-being encompass the intricate interplay of physical, mental, emotional, and spiritual dimensions. By recognizing the multifaceted nature of detoxification, you embark on a transformative journey that nurtures not only your body but also your mind and spirit.

This holistic approach begins with understanding the interconnectedness of these dimensions. The physical body is a temple that houses your consciousness, emotions, and spiritual essence. When you focus solely on physical detoxification, such as through restrictive diets or detox protocols, you may neglect the deeper layers of cleansing that are equally essential.

Mental detoxification involves decluttering your mind, releasing negative thoughts, and cultivating a positive mindset. This can be achieved through practices like meditation, mindfulness, and cognitive-behavioral therapy. By addressing mental blocks and limiting beliefs, you create space for clarity, creativity, and emotional well-being.

Emotional detoxification is about processing and releasing pent-up emotions, traumas, and unresolved issues. This can involve journaling, therapy, or engaging in activities that bring emotional catharsis, such as art, music, or dance. When you allow yourself to feel and heal your emotions, you liberate yourself from their hold on your well-being.

Spiritual detoxification is about connecting with your higher self, finding meaning and purpose in life, and aligning your actions with your core values. This can involve spiritual practices such as meditation, prayer, or connecting with nature. By nurturing your spiritual side, you cultivate a sense of inner peace, tranquility, and a deeper understanding of your place in the universe.

The holistic approach advocated in this book provides a comprehensive roadmap for achieving a balanced and sustainable state of well-being. By addressing the physical, mental, emotional, and spiritual aspects of detoxification, you embark on a profound journey of transformation that brings lasting vitality, clarity, and inner harmony.

Practical Strategies for a Healthier Life

"Detox Diets for the Modern Age" is not just a theoretical exploration of detoxification; it is a practical guide designed to help you implement lasting changes in your life. Each chapter includes actionable tips, recipes, and resources to support you on your journey towards a healthier, toxin-free existence.

Navigating the World of Detox Diets
and Lifestyle Changes

With so much information available on dctox diets and lifestyle changes, it can be challenging to separate fact from fiction. This book aims to cut through the noise and provide you with evidence-based, reliable information to help you make informed decisions about your health. By the end of this book, you will have the knowledge and confidence to embark on a successful detoxification journey and maintain a healthier, more vibrant life in the face of our modern toxic landscape.

Part I: Understanding Detoxification

CHAPTER 1: WHAT IS DETOXIFICATION?

Defining Detoxification in the Modern Context

Detoxification, commonly known as "detox," is a vital process that safeguards the body's health and well-being. In today's world, the importance of detoxification has become paramount due to the prevalence of environmental pollutants, processed food items, and synthetic chemicals that permeate our daily lives. These substances can overwhelm the body's natural detoxification systems, leading to the accumulation of harmful toxins in our tissues and organs, which can potentially trigger a myriad of health concerns.

The detoxification process involves several key steps:

1. **Identification**: The body's defense mechanisms, such as the liver and kidneys, play a crucial role in recognizing and identifying toxic substances that enter the body. This is a complex process that involves various mechanisms, including specialized receptors, enzymes, and transport proteins. Once a toxic substance is identified, the body initiates a cascade of responses to neutralize and eliminate it.

2. **Neutralization**: Once toxic substances are identified, the body employs various mechanisms to neutralize their harmful effects. This can include enzymatic reactions, conjugation with other molecules to form less toxic compounds, and the production of antioxidants to counteract the damaging effects of free radicals. The liver is

the primary organ responsible for neutralizing toxins, but other tissues, such as the kidneys, lungs, and skin, also play a role in this process.

3. **Elimination**: The neutralized toxins are then eliminated from the body through various routes. The kidneys are the primary route of elimination, excreting toxins in the urine. The liver also plays a crucial role by converting toxins into bile, which is excreted through the gastrointestinal tract. The lungs excrete volatile toxins through exhalation, and the skin eliminates toxins through sweat.

The importance of detoxification cannot be overstated. It is a fundamental process that helps protect the body from the damaging effects of toxins, promotes overall health and well-being, and supports the optimal functioning of our organs and systems. By understanding the significance of detoxification, we can make informed choices to reduce our exposure to harmful substances and support our body's natural detoxification processes. This can be achieved by consuming a balanced diet rich in fruits, vegetables, and whole grains, minimizing the intake of processed foods and sugary drinks, engaging in regular exercise, getting adequate sleep, managing stress, and avoiding exposure to environmental toxins as much as possible.

The Science Behind Detoxification: How Your Body Eliminates Toxins

The human body's detoxification process is a vital mechanism that helps maintain overall health and well-being. Several organs and systems work together to identify, break down, and eliminate toxins from the body.

The Liver:

- The liver plays a pivotal role in detoxification by filtering toxins from the bloodstream. Hepatocytes, specialized liver cells, use enzymes to convert these toxins into less harmful substances.

- One of the liver's primary functions is metabolism, which includes breaking down nutrients from food and converting them into energy. During this process, potentially harmful substances can be produced as byproducts. The liver ensures that these substances are processed and detoxified before they can cause harm to the body.

The Kidneys:

- The kidneys are responsible for filtering waste products and excess fluids from the blood. This process, known as glomerular filtration, helps remove toxins, urea, creatinine, and other waste substances.
- The filtered waste products are then concentrated and excreted through urine. The kidneys also help regulate the body's fluid balance and electrolyte levels, which are crucial for overall health.

The Gut:

- The gut, particularly the large intestine, plays a vital role in detoxification through the gut-liver axis. Beneficial bacteria in the gut ferment dietary fiber, producing short-chain fatty acids (SCFAs) such as acetate, propionate, and butyrate.
- SCFAs have various health benefits, including enhancing the liver's detoxification capacity and reducing inflammation. Additionally, the gut microbiome helps break down toxins and prevent their absorption into the bloodstream, supporting the body's detoxification process.

The Skin:

- The skin is the largest organ of the human body and serves as a barrier against external toxins and pathogens. It helps eliminate toxins through sweat, which contains water, electrolytes, and waste products.
- The skin also plays a role in the absorption of certain substances, including topical medications and chemicals

from the environment. Therefore, it's essential to protect the skin from exposure to harmful substances and maintain its integrity as a barrier.

The Lungs:

- The lungs are involved in detoxification through the process of exhalation. When we breathe out, we release carbon dioxide, a waste product of cellular metabolism, and other volatile compounds.
- The lungs also help filter out harmful particles and microbes from the air we breathe, preventing their entry into the bloodstream. This process is important for maintaining respiratory health and supporting the body's detoxification efforts.

Myths and Misconceptions About Detoxification

Despite the growing popularity of detox diets and cleanses, there are many myths and misconceptions surrounding detoxification. Some common myths include:

1. **Myth:** Detox diets are a quick fix for weight loss and health problems.
   Fact: While detox diets may lead to short-term weight loss, they are not a sustainable solution for long-term health and weight management. Detoxification is a gradual process that requires consistent lifestyle changes.
2. **Myth:** You need expensive supplements and products to detoxify your body.
   Fact: While certain supplements can support detoxification, the most effective way to detoxify is through a balanced diet, regular exercise, and healthy lifestyle habits.
3. **Myth:** Detox diets are safe for everyone.
   Fact: Some detox diets can be extreme and may not be suitable for everyone, particularly pregnant

women, children, and individuals with certain health conditions. It's essential to consult with a healthcare professional before starting any detox program.

By understanding the science behind detoxification and dispelling common myths, you can approach detoxification with a more informed and realistic perspective. In the following chapters, we will delve deeper into the various aspects of detoxification, providing you with the knowledge and tools necessary to support your body's natural cleansing processes.

CHAPTER 2: THE MODERN TOXIC LANDSCAPE

The modern world presents a unique set of challenges when it comes to toxin exposure. From the air we breathe to the products we use, toxins are ubiquitous in our environment. Understanding the various sources of toxins and their potential impact on our health is crucial for developing effective detoxification strategies.

Environmental Toxins: Air, Water, and Soil Pollution

Environmental pollution is a significant contributor to the modern toxic burden. Industrial emissions, vehicle exhaust, and the burning of fossil fuels release a wide range of toxins into the air, including particulate matter, volatile organic compounds (VOCs), and heavy metals. These pollutants can be inhaled directly or settle on surfaces, contaminating water and soil.

Water pollution, caused by industrial waste, agricultural runoff, and sewage, exposes us to a variety of toxins, including pesticides, pharmaceuticals, and microplastics. Soil pollution, often the result of improper waste disposal and the use of synthetic fertilizers and pesticides, can lead to the contamination of our food supply.

Toxins in Food: Pesticides, Herbicides, and GMOs

The modern agricultural industry heavily relies on the use of synthetic pesticides and herbicides to control pests and weeds.

These chemicals can remain on or in our food, exposing us to toxins that can accumulate in our bodies over time. Some common pesticides, such as organophosphates, have been linked to neurotoxicity, developmental disorders, and endocrine disruption.

Genetically modified organisms (GMOs) are another potential source of toxins in our food supply. While the long-term health effects of GMOs are still being studied, some research suggests that they may contribute to the development of food allergies, antibiotic resistance, and digestive issues.

Hidden Toxins: Personal Care Products, Cleaning Supplies, and More

Many everyday products, such as cosmetics, toiletries, and cleaning supplies, contain a wide range of synthetic chemicals that can be absorbed through the skin or inhaled.

Phthalates:

- **What they are:** Phthalates are a group of chemicals used to make plastics more flexible and durable. They are also used as solvents (dissolving agents) in many personal care products.
- **Where they're found:** Phthalates are commonly found in perfumes, lotions, shampoos, nail polish, hairspray, and even some children's toys.
- **Health concerns:** Studies have linked phthalates to hormonal disruption, reproductive problems (reduced sperm count, birth defects), and developmental issues in children. Some phthalates are suspected carcinogens.

Parabens:

- **What they are:** Parabens are preservatives used in many cosmetics and personal care products to prevent the growth of bacteria and mold.
- **Where they're found:** Parabens are commonly found

in shampoos, conditioners, lotions, facial cleansers, and makeup.

- **Health concerns:** Parabens can mimic estrogen in the body, potentially disrupting hormonal balance. Some studies have suggested a link between parabens and breast cancer, although more research is needed.

Triclosan:

- **What it is:** Triclosan is an antibacterial and antifungal agent.
- **Where it's found:** Triclosan was once widely used in antibacterial soaps, hand sanitizers, and some toothpastes. However, due to concerns about its safety and effectiveness, it has been banned in many consumer products.
- **Health concerns:** Triclosan has been linked to hormonal disruption and may contribute to the development of antibiotic-resistant bacteria.

Volatile Organic Compounds (VOCs):

- **What they are:** VOCs are a large group of chemicals that easily become gases or vapors at room temperature.
- **Where they're found:** VOCs are found in many household products, including paints, varnishes, cleaning supplies, air fresheners, and even some furniture and building materials.
- **Health concerns:** VOCs can cause a range of health problems, depending on the specific chemical and level of exposure. Short-term effects can include eye, nose, and throat irritation, headaches, and dizziness. Long-term exposure has been linked to cancer, liver and kidney damage, and central nervous system damage.

Reducing Exposure:

- **Read labels carefully:** Look for products labeled "phthalate-free," "paraben-free," and "triclosan-free."
- **Choose fragrance-free products:** Fragrances often contain phthalates and other potentially harmful chemicals.

- **Use natural cleaning products:** Opt for cleaning products made with natural ingredients like vinegar, baking soda, and essential oils.
- **Ventilate your home:** Open windows and use exhaust fans to reduce the concentration of VOCs from paints, cleaning products, and other sources.
- **Research safer alternatives:** Many resources are available online and in stores to help you find safer alternatives to conventional products.

By being mindful of the products you use and making informed choices, you can significantly reduce your exposure to these everyday toxins and protect your health.

The Impact of Technology on Toxicity

The rapid advancement of technology has introduced new sources of toxins into our environment. Electronic devices, such as smartphones, laptops, and televisions, emit electromagnetic fields (EMFs) that can disrupt cellular function and contribute to oxidative stress. The manufacture and disposal of these devices also release toxins into the environment, including heavy metals and flame retardants.

By understanding the various sources of toxins in our modern world, we can take proactive steps to minimize our exposure and support our body's natural detoxification processes. In the next chapter, we will explore how these toxins affect our bodies and the mechanisms through which they contribute to health issues.

CHAPTER 3: HOW TOXINS AFFECT YOUR BODY

Toxins can have a wide range of effects on the human body, from acute reactions to long-term, chronic health issues. Understanding the different types of toxicity and the mechanisms through which toxins impact our health is essential for developing targeted detoxification strategies.

Acute vs. Chronic Toxicity: Understanding the Different Effects

Acute Toxicity

- **Definition:** Acute toxicity results from a single exposure to a high dose of a toxin or multiple exposures over a short period.
- **Examples:** Accidental poisoning, drug overdose, exposure to high levels of pesticides or industrial chemicals.
- **Symptoms:** Symptoms typically appear quickly and can be severe, including headaches, nausea, vomiting, dizziness, skin irritation, respiratory distress, seizures, or even coma and death.
- **Treatment:** Often requires immediate medical attention, including decontamination, supportive care, and administration of antidotes if available.

Chronic Toxicity

- **Definition:** Chronic toxicity results from repeated exposure to low levels of toxins over an extended period, often months or years.
- **Examples:** Long-term exposure to air pollution, heavy metals in food or water, or chemicals in personal care products.
- **Symptoms:** Symptoms may be subtle and nonspecific initially, such as fatigue, headaches, digestive problems, or skin rashes. Over time, chronic toxicity can lead to the development of chronic diseases like cancer, neurological disorders, autoimmune diseases, and cardiovascular problems.
- **Treatment:** Focuses on identifying and eliminating the source of exposure, supporting the body's natural detoxification processes, and managing the symptoms of any resulting health conditions.

The Body's Response to Toxins

The body has several mechanisms to deal with toxins, including:

- **Biotransformation:** The liver and other organs convert toxins into less harmful substances that can be excreted.
- **Excretion:** The kidneys, liver, and intestines eliminate toxins through urine, bile, and feces.
- **Storage:** Some toxins, particularly fat-soluble ones, are stored in fat tissue to minimize their immediate harm. However, this can lead to long-term health problems.

The Importance of Detoxification

Detoxification aims to support the body's natural processes for eliminating toxins and reducing the toxic burden. This can be achieved through dietary changes, lifestyle modifications, and targeted detoxification therapies. By reducing toxin exposure and supporting detoxification, individuals can improve their overall health, prevent chronic diseases, and enhance their body's natural healing abilities.

The Gut-Brain Connection: How Toxins Impact Mental Health

The gut-brain axis is a complex communication network between the digestive system and the central nervous system. Toxins can disrupt this delicate balance, contributing to a range of mental health issues, including:

- **Anxiety and depression:** Toxins can alter neurotransmitter production and function, leading to mood imbalances and emotional distress.
- **Brain fog and cognitive decline:** Exposure to neurotoxins, such as heavy metals, can impair cognitive function, causing memory loss, confusion, and difficulty concentrating.
- **Autism spectrum disorders (ASD):** Some studies suggest that environmental toxins, particularly heavy metals, may contribute to the development of ASD by disrupting neurodevelopment and altering immune function.

Maintaining a healthy gut microbiome through diet, probiotics, and other detoxification strategies can help support the gut-brain connection and promote mental well-being.

The Link Between Toxins and Chronic Diseases

Chronic Toxicity: The Silent Threat to Health

Chronic toxicity, stemming from prolonged exposure to low levels of toxins, poses a significant risk to human health. Unlike acute toxicity, where symptoms are often immediate and severe, chronic toxicity can silently wreak havoc on the body over time. The insidious nature of chronic toxicity makes it a formidable adversary, as its effects may not manifest until significant damage has occurred.

The Culprits:

- **Environmental Toxins:** Persistent organic pollutants (POPs) like pesticides, industrial chemicals, and heavy metals can accumulate in the body over time, gradually impairing organ function and contributing to chronic diseases.
- **Dietary Toxins:** Processed foods, artificial additives, and contaminants in conventionally grown produce can burden the body's detoxification systems and contribute to chronic inflammation and oxidative stress.
- **Lifestyle Factors:** Sedentary behavior, poor sleep, and chronic stress can hinder the body's natural detoxification processes, exacerbating the effects of toxins.

The Consequences:

- **Cardiovascular Disease:** Toxins can promote oxidative stress, inflammation, and the accumulation of arterial plaque, increasing the risk of heart disease, stroke, and other cardiovascular conditions.
- **Cancer:** Many toxins, including pesticides, heavy metals, and industrial chemicals, are known or suspected carcinogens, capable of damaging DNA and promoting the development of various cancers.
- **Autoimmune Disorders:** Toxins can disrupt immune function, triggering an overactive immune response that attacks the body's own tissues, leading to autoimmune diseases like rheumatoid arthritis, lupus, and multiple sclerosis.
- **Endocrine Disruption:** Endocrine-disrupting chemicals (EDCs) found in plastics, pesticides, and personal care products can mimic or block hormones, leading to

imbalances that affect reproductive health, metabolism, and even cancer risk.

- **Neurological Disorders:** Chronic exposure to heavy metals like mercury and lead can damage the nervous system, contributing to cognitive decline, neurodegenerative diseases, and mood disorders.

The Role of Genetics in Detoxification:

Genetic variations play a crucial role in how effectively an individual can detoxify and eliminate toxins. Genes provide the blueprint for enzymes and other proteins involved in detoxification pathways. Variations in these genes, known as polymorphisms, can affect the function of these enzymes, either enhancing or impairing their ability to neutralize and eliminate toxins.

Key Genetic Players:

- **MTHFR Gene:** This gene provides instructions for making an enzyme crucial for methylation, a process involved in detoxification, DNA repair, and neurotransmitter synthesis. Variations in the MTHFR gene can impair methylation and increase susceptibility to heavy metal toxicity, cardiovascular disease, and certain cancers.
- **GST Genes:** Glutathione S-transferase (GST) enzymes play a vital role in phase II detoxification in the liver. Genetic variations in GST genes can affect the body's ability to neutralize and eliminate various toxins, including pesticides and carcinogens.
- **CYP Genes:** Cytochrome P450 (CYP) enzymes are involved in phase I detoxification, where toxins are modified to prepare them for elimination. Genetic variations in CYP genes can influence the rate at which certain toxins are metabolized, affecting an individual's susceptibility to their adverse effects.

Personalized Detoxification:

Understanding one's genetic predispositions can help tailor detoxification strategies to individual needs. For example, individuals with MTHFR polymorphisms may benefit from targeted supplementation to support methylation and detoxification pathways. Similarly, those with variations in GST or CYP genes may need to avoid certain toxins or adopt specific dietary and lifestyle modifications to optimize their detoxification capacity.

By recognizing the interplay between chronic toxicity and genetics, we can develop personalized detoxification approaches that address individual vulnerabilities and promote optimal health. In the next chapter, we will delve deeper into the body's natural detoxification systems and explore how we can support them through diet, lifestyle, and targeted interventions.

CHAPTER 4: YOUR BODY'S NATURAL DETOXIFICATION SYSTEMS

Your body is equipped with a sophisticated network of organs and systems designed to identify, neutralize, and eliminate toxins. By understanding these natural detoxification pathways, you can better support your body's innate ability to cleanse itself.

The Liver: Your Body's Primary Detoxification Organ

The liver is the central hub of detoxification, responsible for breaking down and neutralizing a wide range of toxins. It accomplishes this through a sophisticated two-phase process:

- **Phase I Detoxification:** In this initial phase, the liver employs a group of enzymes called cytochrome P450 to modify toxins. These enzymes make toxins more water-soluble, which is essential for their elimination. However, this process can sometimes create intermediate compounds that are even more reactive and potentially harmful than the original toxins.

- **Phase II Detoxification:** This phase involves neutralizing the reactive intermediate compounds produced in Phase I. The liver attaches molecules like glutathione, sulfate, or glucuronic acid to these compounds, making them less harmful and easier to excrete through urine or bile.

Supporting Liver Health:

To optimize your liver's detoxification capacity, consider the following:

- **Nutrient-Dense Diet:** Consume a diet rich in fruits, vegetables, and whole grains, which provide essential vitamins, minerals, and antioxidants that support liver function.
- **Adequate Hydration:** Drink plenty of water to help flush out toxins and support the liver's filtration processes.
- **Targeted Supplements:** Certain supplements, such as milk thistle, N-acetylcysteine (NAC), and alpha-lipoic acid, have been shown to support liver health and enhance detoxification.

The Kidneys: Filtering Waste and Toxins

The kidneys are the body's filtration system, constantly working to remove waste products and toxins from the blood. They also play a crucial role in maintaining fluid and electrolyte balance, regulating blood pressure, and producing hormones that are essential for overall health.

Supporting Kidney Function:

To keep your kidneys healthy and functioning optimally, consider the following:

- **Stay Hydrated:** Drink plenty of water to help the kidneys flush out waste and toxins efficiently.
- **Limit Processed Foods:** Processed foods are often high in sodium and added sugars, which can burden the kidneys. Opt for whole, unprocessed foods instead.
- **Moderate Protein Intake:** Excessive protein intake can strain the kidneys. Aim for a moderate protein intake from healthy sources like lean meats, fish, legumes, and nuts.

The Gut Microbiome: The Role of Beneficial Bacteria

The gut microbiome, a vast community of trillions of bacteria residing in your digestive tract, plays a crucial role in detoxification. These beneficial bacteria aid in breaking down toxins, preventing their absorption into the bloodstream, and supporting the integrity of the gut lining, which acts as a barrier against harmful substances.

Nurturing Your Gut Microbiome:

To maintain a healthy gut microbiome and enhance detoxification, consider the following:

- **Fiber-Rich Diet:** Consume a diet rich in fruits, vegetables, and whole grains, which provide prebiotic fibers that nourish beneficial gut bacteria.
- **Fermented Foods:** Incorporate fermented foods like yogurt, sauerkraut, kimchi, and kefir, which are natural sources of probiotics (live beneficial bacteria).
- **Probiotic Supplements:** Consider taking probiotic supplements to replenish and diversify your gut microbiome.

The Lymphatic System: Supporting Detoxification

The lymphatic system is a network of vessels, nodes, and organs that helps remove toxins and waste products from the body. It acts as a drainage system, collecting excess fluid and waste from tissues and transporting it back to the bloodstream for filtration and elimination. The lymphatic system also plays a crucial role in immune function, as it houses immune cells that help identify and neutralize harmful substances.

Enhancing Lymphatic Flow:

To support lymphatic flow and enhance detoxification, consider the following:

- **Exercise:** Physical activity, such as brisk walking, jogging, or rebounding, helps stimulate lymphatic flow and promotes the removal of toxins.
- **Massage:** Lymphatic massage, a specialized technique, can manually stimulate lymphatic drainage and improve the removal of waste products.
- **Deep Breathing:** Deep breathing exercises can help activate the lymphatic system by creating pressure changes in the chest and abdomen.

The Skin: Eliminating Toxins Through Sweat

The skin, the body's largest organ, plays a vital role in detoxification by eliminating toxins through sweat. Sweat contains various waste products, including heavy metals, urea, and lactic acid.

Promoting Skin Detoxification:

To support the skin's detoxification function, consider the following:

- **Regular Exercise:** Engaging in physical activity that induces sweating helps eliminate toxins through the skin.
- **Sauna Therapy:** Sauna sessions can promote profuse sweating and enhance the removal of toxins.
- **Dry Brushing:** This practice involves brushing the skin with a natural bristle brush to stimulate lymphatic flow and exfoliate dead skin cells.
- **Hydration:** Drinking plenty of water is essential for supporting sweat production and overall detoxification.

By understanding and supporting the body's natural detoxification systems, you can enhance your overall health, reduce your toxic burden, and promote optimal well-being. Remember, detoxification is an ongoing process, and adopting a holistic approach that encompasses diet, lifestyle, and targeted interventions can empower you to take charge of your health and thrive in the modern world.

Part II: Detoxification for Different Life Stages

CHAPTER 5: DETOX FOR TEENAGERS: BUILDING HEALTHY HABITS

The teenage years are a crucial time for establishing healthy habits that can last a lifetime. By supporting detoxification during this formative period, teenagers can lay the foundation for optimal health and well-being.

Navigating Peer Pressure and Unhealthy Food Choices

Peer pressure and the abundance of processed, nutrient-poor foods can make it challenging for teenagers to maintain a healthy diet. Encouraging them to make informed food choices, pack their own lunches, and engage in meal planning can help them navigate these obstacles.

The Impact of Social Media and Technology on Well-being

Excessive screen time and social media use can contribute to stress, sleep disturbances, and a sedentary lifestyle. Encouraging teenagers to set boundaries around technology use, engage in regular physical activity, and prioritize sleep can support their overall health and detoxification processes.

Building a Healthy Relationship with Food and Exercise

Fostering a positive relationship with food and exercise is essential for long-term health. Encouraging teenagers to view food as nourishment rather than restriction, and to engage in physical activities they enjoy, can help them develop sustainable healthy habits.

Natural Detox Strategies for Teenagers

Some natural detox strategies that can benefit teenagers include:

- Drinking plenty of water to support hydration and waste elimination
- Incorporating nutrient-dense, whole foods into their diet
- Engaging in regular physical activity to promote lymphatic flow and sweating
- Practicing stress-management techniques, such as deep breathing or meditation
- Limiting exposure to environmental toxins, such as those found in personal care products or cleaning supplies

By empowering teenagers with the knowledge and tools to support detoxification, we can help them establish a strong foundation for lifelong health.

CHAPTER 6: DETOX FOR CHILDREN: PROTECTING THEIR GROWING BODIES

Children are especially vulnerable to the harmful effects of toxins, as their developing bodies and brains are more sensitive to environmental insults. Supporting detoxification during childhood is essential for promoting healthy growth and development.

The Vulnerability of Children to Environmental Toxins

Children's rapid growth and development make them more susceptible to the harmful effects of toxins. They also have a higher surface area to body weight ratio, which increases their exposure to toxins in the environment.

Additionally, children's immature detoxification systems may not be able to process and eliminate toxins as effectively as adults, leading to a higher risk of accumulation and potential health issues.

Creating a Safe and Healthy Home Environment

To minimize children's exposure to toxins, it's important to create a safe and healthy home environment. This can be achieved by:

- Using natural, non-toxic cleaning products and personal care items
- Choosing organic, whole foods whenever possible
- Filtering air and water to reduce exposure to pollutants
- Avoiding the use of pesticides and herbicides in the home and garden
- Opting for natural, non-toxic building materials and furnishings

Choosing Safe Toys and Products for Children

Many children's toys and products can contain harmful toxins, such as lead, phthalates, and bisphenol A (BPA). To protect children from these toxins, it's important to:

- Choose toys made from natural, non-toxic materials like wood, cotton, or wool
- Avoid plastic toys, especially those made from PVC or containing phthalates
- Opt for BPA-free bottles, sippy cups, and food storage containers
- Read labels carefully and research products before purchasing

Nutritional Guidelines for Children's Detoxification

Supporting children's detoxification processes through nutrition is essential for their overall health and development. Some key nutritional guidelines include:

- Providing a balanced diet rich in fruits, vegetables, whole grains, and lean proteins
- Limiting processed foods, refined sugars, and artificial additives
- Ensuring adequate hydration through water and other unsweetened beverages
- Incorporating nutrient-dense superfoods, such as berries, leafy greens, and nuts

- Considering age-appropriate supplements, such as omega-3 fatty acids and probiotics, under the guidance of a healthcare professional

By prioritizing a safe, healthy environment and providing optimal nutrition, we can support children's natural detoxification processes and promote their long-term health and well-being.

CHAPTER 7: DETOX FOR ADULTS: ADDRESSING SPECIFIC CONCERNS

Adults face unique challenges when it comes to detoxification, as years of exposure to toxins, combined with the stresses of modern life, can take a toll on their health. Addressing specific concerns and tailoring detoxification strategies to individual needs is essential for promoting optimal wellness.

Detoxification for Stress and Burnout

Chronic stress and burnout can impair the body's natural detoxification processes, leading to an accumulation of toxins and an increased risk of health issues. To support detoxification during times of stress, consider:

- Practicing stress-management techniques, such as meditation, deep breathing, or yoga
- Prioritizing sleep and maintaining a consistent sleep schedule
- Engaging in regular physical activity to promote circulation and lymphatic flow
- Incorporating adaptogenic herbs, such as ashwagandha or rhodiola, to support the body's stress response
- Seeking support from friends, family, or mental health

professionals when needed

Detoxification for Hormonal Imbalances

Hormonal imbalances can be exacerbated by exposure to toxins, particularly endocrine-disrupting chemicals (EDCs). To support detoxification and promote hormonal balance:

- Minimize exposure to EDCs by choosing natural, non-toxic personal care and household products
- Support liver function through a nutrient-dense diet and targeted supplements, such as milk thistle or dandelion root
- Incorporate hormone-balancing foods, such as cruciferous vegetables, flaxseeds, and fermented soy products
- Consider working with a healthcare professional to assess hormone levels and develop a personalized treatment plan

Detoxification for Fertility and Reproductive Health

Exposure to toxins can impact fertility and reproductive health in both men and women. To support detoxification and promote optimal reproductive function:

- Minimize exposure to toxins, particularly those known to impact reproductive health, such as phthalates and heavy metals
- Support detoxification pathways through a nutrient-rich diet and targeted supplements, such as folate, zinc, and antioxidants
- Incorporate fertility-boosting foods, such as leafy greens, omega-3-rich fish, and nuts
- Address underlying health conditions that may impact fertility, such as polycystic ovary syndrome (PCOS) or endometriosis

Detoxification for Chronic Diseases

Chronic diseases, such as autoimmune disorders, cardiovascular disease, and cancer, can be influenced by toxin exposure and impaired detoxification processes. To support detoxification in the context of chronic disease:

- Work with a healthcare professional to identify potential toxin exposures and develop a personalized detoxification plan
- Focus on an anti-inflammatory, nutrient-dense diet rich in fruits, vegetables, whole grains, and healthy fats
- Consider targeted supplements, such as glutathione, curcumin, or omega-3 fatty acids, to support detoxification and reduce inflammation
- Engage in gentle physical activity, such as walking or swimming, to promote circulation and lymphatic flow
- Prioritize stress management and self-care practices to support overall health and well-being

By addressing specific concerns and tailoring detoxification strategies to individual needs, adults can optimize their health and promote long-term vitality in the face of the modern toxic landscape.

CHAPTER 8: DETOX FOR THE ELDERLY: MAINTAINING VITALITY

As we age, our bodies' natural detoxification processes may become less efficient, making it increasingly important to support these systems through targeted interventions. By prioritizing detoxification in the elderly, we can help maintain vitality and promote healthy aging.

Age-Related Changes in Detoxification Capacity

Several factors can contribute to a decline in detoxification capacity as we age:

- Decreased liver and kidney function, leading to slower processing and elimination of toxins
- Reduced glutathione levels, a key antioxidant involved in detoxification
- Decreased digestive enzyme production, impacting the body's ability to break down and absorb nutrients
- Chronic inflammation and oxidative stress, which can impair detoxification pathways

By understanding these age-related changes, we can develop targeted strategies to support detoxification in the elderly.

Detoxification for Cognitive Health and Memory

Supporting detoxification can be particularly important for maintaining cognitive health and memory as we age. To promote brain health through detoxification:

- Focus on a nutrient-dense, anti-inflammatory diet rich in omega-3 fatty acids, antioxidants, and B vitamins
- Incorporate brain-boosting foods, such as blueberries, turmeric, and leafy greens
- Consider targeted supplements, such as acetyl-L-carnitine, ginkgo biloba, or phosphatidylserine, to support cognitive function
- Engage in regular physical activity and mentally stimulating activities to promote brain health
- Prioritize sleep and stress management to support overall brain function

Detoxification for Joint Health and Mobility

Toxin exposure and impaired detoxification can contribute to inflammation and joint health issues in the elderly. To support joint health through detoxification:

- Incorporate anti-inflammatory foods, such as turmeric, ginger, and omega-3-rich fish
- Limit processed foods, refined sugars, and unhealthy fats that can promote inflammation
- Consider supplements like glucosamine, chondroitin, or MSM to support joint health
- Engage in low-impact, joint-friendly exercises, such as swimming, tai chi, or yoga
- Maintain a healthy weight to reduce stress on joints

Nutritional Considerations for Seniors

Optimal nutrition is essential for supporting detoxification and overall health in the elderly. Some key nutritional considerations include:

- Ensuring adequate protein intake to support muscle mass and immune function
- Focusing on nutrient-dense foods to compensate for reduced caloric needs
- Incorporating healthy fats, such as omega-3s and monounsaturated fats, to support brain and joint health
- Staying well-hydrated to support waste elimination and overall bodily functions
- Considering targeted supplements, such as vitamin D, B12, and probiotics, to address common nutrient deficiencies and support gut health

By prioritizing detoxification and optimal nutrition, we can help the elderly maintain vitality, cognitive function, and joint health in the face of age-related challenges.

Part III: Detoxification Strategies

CHAPTER 9:
DETOX DIETS: THE FOUNDATION OF DETOXIFICATION

Detox diets form the foundation of many detoxification programs, focusing on nutrient-dense, whole foods that support the body's natural cleansing processes. By understanding the principles and types of detox diets, you can choose the approach that best suits your individual needs and goals.

Principles of a Detox Diet

While detox diets can vary in their specific guidelines, they generally adhere to a few key principles:

- Emphasizing whole, minimally processed foods, such as fruits, vegetables, whole grains, lean proteins, and healthy fats
- Eliminating or minimizing common allergens and inflammatory foods, such as gluten, dairy, soy, and processed sugars
- Incorporating detoxifying foods and beverages, such as leafy greens, cruciferous vegetables, and herbal teas
- Promoting adequate hydration through water, herbal teas, and other non-caffeinated beverages
- Supporting the body's natural detoxification processes

through targeted nutrients and phytochemicals

Types of Detox Diets: Choosing the Right One for You

- **Juice Cleanses:** These diets involve consuming only fruit and vegetable juices for a set period, typically ranging from a few days to a week or longer.
    - **Pros:** Provides a concentrated dose of vitamins, minerals, and enzymes; may help reduce inflammation and improve digestion.
    - **Cons:** Lacks fiber and protein, which are essential for satiety and overall health; can be difficult to sustain long-term; may lead to nutrient deficiencies if not done properly.
- **Intermittent Fasting:** This approach involves cycling between periods of eating and voluntary fasting on a regular schedule. Popular methods include the 16/8 method (16 hours of fasting followed by an 8-hour eating window) and alternate-day fasting.
    - **Pros:** Promotes cellular repair and autophagy (the body's process of cleaning out damaged cells); may improve insulin sensitivity and reduce inflammation; can be a sustainable approach for some individuals.
    - **Cons:** May not be suitable for everyone, especially those with certain medical conditions; can be challenging to adapt to initially; may lead to side effects like headaches or fatigue in the beginning.
- **Whole Foods Detox:** This approach focuses on consuming whole, unprocessed foods like fruits, vegetables, whole grains, legumes, nuts, and seeds while eliminating processed foods, refined sugars, artificial ingredients, and common allergens.
    - **Pros:** Provides a wide range of nutrients and fiber; supports gut health and the microbiome; can be a sustainable, long-term approach to detoxification and overall health.

     ○   **Cons:** May require more meal planning and preparation; can be challenging to eliminate all processed foods from the diet; may not be as restrictive as other detox diets, which some individuals may prefer.

When choosing a detox diet, it's crucial to consider your individual health status, goals, and preferences. Consult with a healthcare professional or registered dietitian before starting any new dietary regimen, especially if you have any underlying health conditions or concerns. They can help you determine the most suitable and safe approach for your specific needs.

Foods to Include and Avoid

When following a detox diet, focus on incorporating the following foods:

- Leafy greens and cruciferous vegetables, such as kale, spinach, broccoli, and cauliflower
- Antioxidant-rich fruits, like berries, citrus fruits, and pomegranates
- Whole grains, such as quinoa, brown rice, and oats
- Lean proteins, including organic poultry, wild-caught fish, and legumes
- Healthy fats, such as avocados, nuts, seeds, and olive oil
- Detoxifying herbs and spices, like turmeric, ginger, garlic, and cilantro

Avoid or minimize the following foods during a detox diet:

- Processed and packaged foods, including snack foods and fast food
- Refined sugars and artificial sweeteners
- Unhealthy fats, such as trans fats and partially hydrogenated oils
- Alcohol and caffeine
- Common allergens and inflammatory foods, such as gluten, dairy, and soy (if sensitive)

Meal Planning and Recipes

To make your detox diet more manageable and enjoyable, consider the following meal planning tips:

- Plan your meals and snacks in advance to ensure you have the necessary ingredients on hand
- Prepare larger batches of meals to have leftovers for busy days
- Incorporate a variety of colors, textures, and flavors to keep your meals interesting and satisfying
- Experiment with new recipes and ingredients to expand your culinary horizons

Here are a few simple, detox-friendly recipes to get you started:

1. Green Smoothie: Blend 1 cup spinach, 1 cup kale, 1 banana, 1 cup frozen berries, 1 tbsp chia seeds, and 1 cup unsweetened almond milk until smooth.
2. Quinoa Salad: Combine 1 cup cooked quinoa, 1/2 cup diced cucumber, 1/2 cup cherry tomatoes, 1/4 cup chopped parsley, and 1/4 cup diced red onion. Drizzle with olive oil and lemon juice, and season with salt and pepper to taste.
3. Baked Salmon with Asparagus: Season a 4 oz salmon fillet with salt, pepper, and lemon juice. Place on a baking sheet lined with parchment paper, and surround with 1 cup of trimmed asparagus spears. Bake at 400°F for 12-15 minutes, or until the salmon is cooked through and the asparagus is tender.

By incorporating a variety of nutrient-dense, whole foods and planning your meals in advance, you can create a sustainable and effective detox diet that supports your body's natural cleansing processes.

CHAPTER 10: SUPPLEMENTS AND HERBS FOR DETOXIFICATION

While a nutrient-dense, whole foods diet forms the foundation of detoxification, targeted supplements and herbs can provide additional support for your body's cleansing processes. By understanding the key nutrients and herbal allies that aid detoxification, you can create a comprehensive approach to supporting your health and well-being.

Essential Vitamins and Minerals for Detoxification

Certain vitamins and minerals play crucial roles in supporting the body's detoxification pathways. Some of the most important include:

- **B vitamins:** B vitamins, particularly B6, B12, and folate, are essential for the proper function of the liver's detoxification enzymes. They also support energy production and help manage stress, which can impact detoxification processes.

- **Vitamin C:** This potent antioxidant helps neutralize free radicals and supports the production of glutathione, a key compound in the body's detoxification pathways. Vitamin C also enhances immune function and aids in the elimination of heavy metals.

- **Vitamin E:** Another powerful antioxidant, vitamin E helps protect cell membranes from oxidative damage and supports the body's natural detoxification processes.
- **Magnesium:** This essential mineral is involved in over 300 enzymatic reactions in the body, including those related to detoxification. Magnesium helps support energy production, relaxation, and regular bowel movements, which are crucial for eliminating toxins.
- **Zinc:** Zinc is a key component of many detoxification enzymes and helps support immune function. It also plays a role in the production of metallothionein, a protein that binds to heavy metals and aids in their elimination.

Herbal Allies for Detoxification

Herbal supplements can provide targeted support for the body's detoxification processes. Some of the most effective herbs for detoxification include:

- **Milk thistle:** This herb is renowned for its liver-supportive properties. Silymarin, the active compound in milk thistle, helps protect liver cells from damage and supports the organ's natural detoxification processes.
- **Dandelion root:** Dandelion root is a gentle diuretic that helps support kidney function and the elimination of toxins through urine. It also aids in liver detoxification and promotes digestive health.
- **Burdock root:** This herb is known for its blood-purifying properties and helps support the body's natural detoxification processes. Burdock root also aids in digestion and supports skin health.
- **Turmeric:** Curcumin, the active compound in turmeric, is a potent anti-inflammatory and antioxidant. It helps support liver function, aids in the production of bile, and enhances the body's natural detoxification processes.
- **Green tea:** Rich in antioxidants called catechins, green tea helps protect cells from oxidative damage and supports

the body's natural detoxification processes. It also provides a gentle energy boost and aids in weight management.

Choosing High-Quality Supplements

When selecting supplements for detoxification, it's crucial to choose high-quality products from reputable brands. Look for supplements that:

- Are free from artificial additives, fillers, and binders
- Use high-quality, bioavailable forms of nutrients
- Are third-party tested for purity and potency
- Provide transparent labeling and dosage instructions

It's also essential to consult with a healthcare professional before starting any new supplement regimen, particularly if you have a pre-existing health condition or are taking medications.

Safety Considerations and Potential Interactions

While supplements and herbs can be powerful allies in detoxification, it's important to be aware of potential safety considerations and interactions:

- Some supplements and herbs can interact with medications or exacerbate certain health conditions. Always consult with a healthcare professional before starting a new supplement regimen.
- Pregnant and breastfeeding women should exercise caution when using supplements and herbs, as some may not be safe for use during these life stages.
- Certain supplements and herbs can cause side effects, such as digestive discomfort, headaches, or allergic reactions. Start with low doses and monitor your body's response.
- Be mindful of the quality and source of your supplements and herbs to avoid contamination or adulteration.

By incorporating targeted supplements and herbs into your detoxification plan, you can provide additional support for your body's natural cleansing processes. However, remember that supplements should be used in conjunction with a nutrient-dense, whole foods diet and healthy lifestyle practices for optimal results.

CHAPTER 11: LIFESTYLE PRACTICES FOR DETOXIFICATION

In addition to diet and supplements, certain lifestyle practices can significantly support your body's natural detoxification processes. By incorporating these practices into your daily routine, you can create a holistic approach to detoxification that promotes overall health and well-being.

Exercise: Boosting Circulation and Lymphatic Flow

Regular exercise is a powerful tool for supporting detoxification, as it helps:

- Increase circulation, which allows nutrients to be delivered to cells and waste products to be removed more efficiently
- Stimulate lymphatic flow, which is crucial for transporting toxins and waste products out of the body
- Promote sweating, which allows toxins to be eliminated through the skin
- Reduce inflammation, which can impair detoxification processes
- Manage stress, which can negatively impact the body's natural cleansing mechanisms

Aim to incorporate a variety of exercises into your routine, including cardiovascular activities, strength training, and flexibility exercises. Find activities that you enjoy and that fit your fitness level to ensure long-term adherence.

Sauna Therapy: Sweating Out Toxins

Sauna therapy, or hyperthermia, is a powerful detoxification tool that involves exposing the body to high temperatures to promote sweating. Benefits of sauna therapy include:

- Promoting the elimination of toxins, such as heavy metals and chemicals, through sweat
- Improving circulation and oxygenation of tissues
- Supporting relaxation and stress reduction
- Enhancing immune function

When using a sauna for detoxification, start with short sessions (5-10 minutes) and gradually increase the duration as your body adjusts. Be sure to stay well-hydrated and listen to your body's signals to avoid overheating or discomfort.

Dry Brushing: Stimulating Lymphatic Drainage

Dry brushing is a simple and effective technique for supporting the body's natural detoxification processes. This practice involves using a soft-bristled brush to gently massage the skin in circular motions, starting at the feet and moving towards the heart. Benefits of dry brushing include:

- Stimulating lymphatic flow, which helps remove toxins and waste products from the body
- Exfoliating the skin, which allows it to better eliminate toxins through sweat
- Improving circulation, which supports nutrient delivery and waste removal
- Promoting relaxation and stress reduction

To practice dry brushing, use a natural-bristled brush and perform the technique on dry skin before showering. Be gentle, especially on sensitive areas, and avoid brushing over broken skin or irritated areas.

Hydrotherapy: Supporting Detoxification Through Water

Hydrotherapy involves the use of water, in various temperatures and forms, to support the body's natural healing and detoxification processes. Some simple hydrotherapy techniques include:

- **Contrast showers:** Alternating between hot and cold water in the shower can help stimulate circulation, boost immune function, and promote detoxification.
- **Epsom salt baths:** Soaking in a warm bath with Epsom salts (magnesium sulfate) can help draw toxins out of the body, support relaxation, and ease muscle tension.
- **Hydration:** Drinking plenty of clean, filtered water throughout the day is essential for supporting the body's natural detoxification processes and promoting the elimination of toxins through urine and sweat.

When using hydrotherapy techniques, be mindful of your body's response and adjust the temperature and duration as needed to ensure comfort and safety.

Mindfulness and Stress Reduction Techniques

Chronic stress can impair the body's natural detoxification processes, making stress management an essential component of any detoxification plan. Some effective stress reduction techniques include:

- **Meditation:** Regular meditation practice can help calm the mind, reduce stress, and promote relaxation, which supports the body's natural healing and detoxification processes.
- **Deep breathing:** Practicing deep, diaphragmatic breathing can help reduce stress, oxygenate the body, and support detoxification through the lungs.
- **Yoga:** This ancient practice combines physical postures, breathing techniques, and meditation to promote relaxation,

reduce stress, and support overall health and well-being.

- **Time in nature:** Spending time outdoors, surrounded by natural elements, can help reduce stress, promote relaxation, and support the body's natural detoxification processes.

Incorporating these lifestyle practices into your daily routine can help create a comprehensive approach to detoxification that supports your body's natural cleansing processes and promotes overall health and well-being. Remember to start slowly, listen to your body's signals, and consult with a healthcare professional if you have any concerns or pre-existing health conditions.

CHAPTER 12: DETOXIFICATION FOR SPECIFIC CONDITIONS

While detoxification can benefit overall health and well-being, certain conditions may warrant a more targeted approach. In this chapter, we'll explore specific detoxification strategies for heavy metal toxicity, chemical exposures, and gut health issues.

Heavy Metal Detoxification

Heavy metals, such as mercury, lead, arsenic, and cadmium, can accumulate in the body over time, leading to a range of health issues. Symptoms of heavy metal toxicity may include fatigue, headaches, cognitive dysfunction, and digestive disturbances. To support heavy metal detoxification:

- Identify and minimize exposure to sources of heavy metals, such as certain types of fish, contaminated water, and industrial pollutants.
- Support the body's natural detoxification processes through a nutrient-dense, whole foods diet rich in antioxidants, fiber, and essential minerals.
- Consider targeted supplements, such as cilantro, chlorella, and modified citrus pectin, which can help bind to heavy metals and support their elimination from the body.
- Work with a qualified healthcare professional to assess your heavy metal burden and develop a personalized detoxification plan, which may include chelation therapy in

severe cases.

Mercury

Mercury is a toxic heavy metal that can accumulate in the body through exposure to contaminated seafood, dental amalgams, and certain industrial processes. To support mercury detoxification:

- Minimize consumption of high-mercury fish, such as shark, swordfish, and tuna.
- Consider having mercury-containing dental amalgams safely removed by a biological dentist.
- Support glutathione production through a diet rich in sulfur-containing foods, such as garlic, onions, and cruciferous vegetables.
- Consider supplements like alpha-lipoic acid, N-acetylcysteine, and selenium, which support mercury detoxification and binding.

Lead

Lead exposure can occur through contaminated water, soil, and older lead-based paints. To support lead detoxification:

- Test your home for lead-based paint and take appropriate measures to minimize exposure, especially if you have young children.
- Filter your drinking water to remove lead and other contaminants.
- Support calcium and iron intake through diet or supplementation, as these minerals can help reduce lead absorption.
- Consider supplements like vitamin C, garlic, and cilantro, which may help support lead detoxification.

Arsenic

Arsenic exposure can occur through contaminated water, certain foods (such as rice), and industrial processes. To support arsenic detoxification:

- Test your drinking water for arsenic and use a filtration system if necessary.
- Vary your grain choices and rinse rice thoroughly before cooking to minimize arsenic exposure.
- Support methylation processes through a diet rich in B vitamins, particularly folate, B6, and B12.
- Consider supplements like spirulina, chlorella, and alpha-lipoic acid, which may help support arsenic detoxification.

Cadmium

Cadmium exposure can occur through cigarette smoke, contaminated water, and certain industrial processes. To support cadmium detoxification:

- Avoid or quit smoking, as tobacco is a significant source of cadmium exposure.
- Minimize consumption of organ meats, as they can accumulate higher levels of cadmium.
- Support zinc and calcium intake through diet or supplementation, as these minerals can help reduce cadmium absorption.
- Consider supplements like vitamin C, milk thistle, and cilantro, which may help support cadmium detoxification.

Chemical Detoxification

Exposure to various chemicals, such as pesticides, herbicides, plasticizers, and mold toxins, can burden the body's detoxification systems and contribute to health issues. To support chemical detoxification:

- Minimize exposure to chemicals by choosing organic foods, using natural cleaning and personal care products, and avoiding plastics when possible.
- Support the body's natural detoxification processes through a nutrient-dense, whole foods diet rich in antioxidants and

fiber.

- Consider targeted supplements, such as glutathione, milk thistle, and green tea extract, which can help support the liver's detoxification pathways.
- Work with a qualified healthcare professional to assess your chemical burden and develop a personalized detoxification plan.

Pesticides and Herbicides

Pesticides and herbicides are widely used in conventional agriculture and can accumulate in the body over time. To support detoxification from these chemicals:

- Choose organic produce whenever possible, especially for items on the "Dirty Dozen" list, which tend to have higher pesticide residues.
- Thoroughly wash all produce, even organic items, to remove surface residues.
- Support glutathione production through a diet rich in sulfur-containing foods, such as garlic, onions, and cruciferous vegetables.
- Consider supplements like milk thistle, dandelion root, and cilantro, which may help support pesticide and herbicide detoxification.

Phthalates and BPA

Phthalates and bisphenol A (BPA) are common plasticizers found in many consumer products, including food packaging, personal care items, and toys. To support detoxification from these chemicals:

- Minimize your use of plastic food containers and choose glass, stainless steel, or ceramic options instead.
- Avoid heating food in plastic containers or covered with plastic wrap.
- Choose personal care products that are labeled "phthalate-free" and "BPA-free."

- Support the body's natural detoxification processes through a diet rich in fiber, which can help bind to phthalates and BPA and promote their elimination.

Mold and Mycotoxins

Exposure to mold and mycotoxins can occur in water-damaged buildings and contribute to a range of health issues, including respiratory problems, neurological symptoms, and immune dysfunction. To support detoxification from mold and mycotoxins:

- Identify and address any sources of mold in your home or workplace, working with a qualified remediation professional if necessary.
- Use air filtration systems with HEPA filters to help remove mold spores and mycotoxins from indoor air.
- Support the body's natural detoxification processes through a diet rich in antioxidants, particularly vitamin C and glutathione.
- Consider targeted supplements, such as activated charcoal, bentonite clay, and cholestyramine, which can help bind to mycotoxins and support their elimination from the body.

Detoxification for Gut Health

The gut plays a crucial role in the body's overall detoxification processes, and imbalances in gut health can contribute to a range of health issues. Common gut health concerns that may benefit from targeted detoxification support include:

Candida Overgrowth

Candida is a type of yeast that naturally occurs in the gut, but overgrowth can lead to digestive issues, fatigue, and other symptoms. To support detoxification and balance of Candida:

- Follow an anti-Candida diet, which typically involves eliminating sugar, refined carbohydrates, and fermented foods while focusing on nutrient-dense, whole foods.

- Consider targeted supplements, such as caprylic acid, oregano oil, and probiotics, which can help support the balance of gut flora and control Candida overgrowth.
- Support the body's natural detoxification processes through a diet rich in fiber and antioxidants.

Parasites

Parasitic infections can contribute to a range of digestive and systemic symptoms and may require targeted detoxification support. To address parasitic infections:

- Work with a qualified healthcare professional to identify the specific parasite and develop an appropriate treatment plan, which may include antiparasitic medications or herbs.
- Support the body's natural detoxification processes through a nutrient-dense, whole foods diet rich in fiber, antioxidants, and anti-inflammatory compounds.
- Consider targeted supplements, such as oregano oil, garlic, and wormwood, which may help support the elimination of parasites.

Leaky Gut Syndrome

Leaky gut syndrome, scientifically referred to as increased intestinal permeability, is a condition characterized by the weakening of the intestinal lining. This weakening allows substances, such as toxins and partially digested food particles, to pass through the intestines and enter the bloodstream. This incursion can lead to various health issues, including systemic inflammation, immune dysfunction, and a host of chronic diseases. Understanding the complexity of leaky gut and the strategies to support its healing is critical for restoring optimal health.

Anti-inflammatory Diet

One of the foundational strategies for addressing leaky gut syndrome involves adopting an anti-inflammatory diet. This diet focuses on eliminating common dietary triggers known to exacerbate inflammation and intestinal permeability. Foods such as gluten, dairy, and highly processed foods contain components that can irritate the gut lining and should be avoided.

Importance of Whole Foods

Simultaneously, emphasizing nutrient-dense, whole foods is vital. These foods provide the essential nutrients needed to support the healing and fortification of the gut lining. Whole foods, rich in antioxidants, vitamins, and minerals, can help reduce inflammation and promote a healthy gut environment.

Targeted Supplementation

To further support the healing of leaky gut, certain targeted supplements can be beneficial:

L-glutamine: An amino acid that is crucial for the repair and regeneration of the intestinal lining. L-glutamine serves as a primary fuel source for the cells in the gut and can help strengthen the barrier function of the intestines.

Collagen peptides: These provide the necessary building blocks for repairing the connective tissue in the gut lining, improving its structural integrity.

Zinc carnosine: A compound known to support the gut's mucosal defense mechanisms, helping to reduce permeability and inflammation.

Gut-Healing Foods

Incorporating specific gut-healing foods into the diet is also essential:

Bone broth: Rich in collagen, gelatin, and various amino acids, bone broth can help heal the gut lining and reduce intestinal inflammation.

Fermented vegetables: Foods like sauerkraut and kimchi are

excellent sources of probiotics, beneficial bacteria that play a critical role in maintaining gut health and balance.

Prebiotic-rich foods: Foods high in prebiotics, such as garlic, onions, and asparagus, feed the beneficial bacteria in the gut, promoting a healthy microbiome.

Professional Guidance

While these dietary and supplemental strategies are valuable, it's important to address any underlying factors contributing to leaky gut syndrome. Chronic stress, bacterial overgrowth (such as small intestinal bacterial overgrowth, or SIBO), and infections can significantly impact gut health. Working with a qualified healthcare professional is crucial to identify these underlying issues and develop a comprehensive, personalized plan. A healthcare provider can offer guidance on diagnostic testing, lifestyle modifications, and further individualized treatment strategies to support detoxification and healing.

Personalized Plan

Every individual's experience with leaky gut syndrome is unique, and thus, the approach to healing should be personalized. A qualified healthcare professional can help tailor a plan that considers your specific health concerns, dietary preferences, and lifestyle factors. This personalized plan is not only more effective but also sustainable in the long term.

Part IV: Maintaining a Detoxified Lifestyle

CHAPTER 13: CREATING A TOXIN-FREE HOME ENVIRONMENT

Creating a toxin-free home environment is an essential aspect of maintaining a detoxified lifestyle. By minimizing your exposure to harmful chemicals and pollutants in your living space, you can support your body's natural detoxification processes and promote overall health and well-being.

Choosing Non-Toxic Cleaning Products

Many conventional cleaning products contain harsh chemicals that can contribute to indoor air pollution and increase your toxic burden. To create a safer, more natural home environment:

- Opt for non-toxic, eco-friendly cleaning products that are free from harmful chemicals, such as phthalates, ammonia, and chlorine bleach.
- Make your own cleaning solutions using simple, natural ingredients like white vinegar, baking soda, and essential oils.
- Use microfiber cloths or reusable, washable cleaning tools instead of disposable options to minimize waste and exposure to chemicals.

Purifying Indoor Air

Let's delve deep into the nuances of the statement that "Indoor air can be more polluted than outdoor air," unraveling the complexities and providing a comprehensive understanding, alongside strategies to combat this issue.

Understanding Indoor Air Pollution

Firstly, it's imperative to grasp the counterintuitive notion that the air within our homes and workplaces can be more contaminated than the air outside. This is primarily due to the lack of circulation, which allows pollutants to accumulate over time. The sources of these pollutants are manifold:

Furniture and Carpets: These can release volatile organic compounds (VOCs), formaldehyde, flame retardants, and other harmful chemicals into the air. Over time, these substances off-gas from their surfaces into the indoor environment.

Electronic Devices: Items such as printers, computers, and televisions can emit particulate matter and VOCs, contributing to the indoor pollution load.

Building Materials: Paints, solvents, and other construction materials can also off-gas VOCs and other pollutants into the air.

Strategies for Improving Indoor Air Quality

Improving indoor air quality necessitates a multifaceted approach, addressing both the reduction of pollutant sources and the purification of the air that circulates within indoor environments.

1. Air Purifiers with HEPA Filters

Mechanism: High-Efficiency Particulate Air (HEPA) filters work by forcing air through a fine mesh that traps harmful particles such as pollen, dust mites, tobacco smoke, and particulate matter.

Effectiveness: HEPA filters are highly effective in removing airborne pollutants. However, it's crucial to choose an air purifier sized appropriately for the room and to regularly replace the filters as per the manufacturer's recommendations.

2. Incorporating Air-Purifying Plants

Functionality: Certain plants have been shown to absorb toxic substances from the air through the process of phytoremediation. For instance, spider plants are effective at removing carbon monoxide and xylene, peace lilies can absorb benzene, and snake plants are known for their ability to purify the air by absorbing toxins and releasing oxygen at night.

Consideration: While plants can contribute to cleaner air, it's important to understand their limitations and not rely solely on them for air purification.

3. Ensuring Adequate Ventilation

Importance: Proper ventilation is crucial for diluting and removing indoor pollutants. This can be achieved by opening windows to allow for the exchange of indoor and outdoor air and using fans to enhance circulation.

Balance: It's essential to strike a balance between ventilating and maintaining energy efficiency, especially in extreme weather conditions.

4. Choosing Low-VOC or Zero-VOC Products

Preventive Measure: Selecting paints, furniture, and carpets that are labeled as low-VOC or zero-VOC can significantly reduce the amount of harmful chemicals released into your indoor environment.

Awareness: Becoming aware of the materials and products that contribute to indoor pollution is the first step in making healthier choices for your indoor spaces.

Understanding the sources and consequences of indoor air pollution is pivotal in taking proactive steps to mitigate its impact on our health. By integrating air purifiers, incorporating air-purifying plants, ensuring adequate ventilation, and choosing low-emission products, we can significantly improve the quality of the air we breathe indoors. It's a holistic approach that requires awareness, action, and continuous effort to maintain a healthy indoor environment.

Filtering Water

Drinking water can contain a variety of contaminants, including heavy metals, pesticides, and chlorine byproducts. To ensure your water is as clean and toxin-free as possible:

- Install a high-quality water filtration system, such as a reverse osmosis or activated carbon filter, to remove contaminants from your drinking water.
- Use a shower filter to minimize exposure to chlorine and other chemicals that can be absorbed through the skin and inhaled in steam.
- Avoid storing or heating water in plastic containers, which can leach chemicals like BPA and phthalates into your water.

Minimizing Electromagnetic Radiation

Electromagnetic fields (EMFs) from electronic devices and wireless networks can potentially disrupt the body's natural processes and contribute to oxidative stress. To minimize your exposure to EMFs:

- Keep electronic devices, such as cell phones and laptops, away from your body when not in use, especially while sleeping.
- Use wired connections instead of Wi-Fi or Bluetooth when possible, particularly for devices you use frequently or for extended periods.
- Consider installing EMF-shielding materials, such as conductive paints or fabrics, in your home or workspace to reduce overall EMF exposure.

- Take regular breaks from electronic devices and spend time in nature to help balance the body's natural electromagnetic fields.

By implementing these strategies for creating a toxin-free home environment, you can support your body's natural detoxification processes and promote long-term health and well-being.

CHAPTER 14: CHOOSING SAFE AND EFFECTIVE DETOX PRODUCTS

When embarking on a detoxification journey, it's essential to choose safe and effective products that support your body's natural cleansing processes. With the vast array of detox supplements and programs available, it can be challenging to navigate the options and make informed decisions.

Evaluating Detox Supplements and Programs

The market for detox supplements and programs is vast and often confusing. To make informed decisions and safeguard your health, it's crucial to approach these products with a discerning eye. Here's a comprehensive guide to evaluating detox supplements and programs:

Ingredients: The Cornerstone of Safety and Efficacy

- **Prioritize natural ingredients:** Look for supplements and programs that utilize natural ingredients with well-established detoxification properties. These may include:
  - **Milk thistle:** A powerful herb that supports liver function and detoxification.
  - **Glutathione:** A master antioxidant that helps

neutralize harmful substances.

- o **Chlorella:** A type of algae rich in chlorophyll, which binds to heavy metals and aids in their elimination.
- o **Activated charcoal:** A porous substance that can adsorb toxins in the gut.
- o **Fiber:** Essential for promoting regular bowel movements and eliminating waste products.
- **Avoid synthetic additives:** Steer clear of products containing artificial colors, flavors, sweeteners, fillers, and preservatives, as these can burden the liver and other detoxification organs.
- **Research individual ingredients:** Thoroughly research each ingredient listed on the label to understand its potential benefits and risks. Consult with a healthcare professional if you have any concerns.

Dosage: Finding the Right Balance

- **Follow recommended dosages:** Adhere to the recommended dosages provided on the product label or by a healthcare professional. Excessively high doses can be harmful and may not necessarily lead to better results.
- **Consider individual needs:** Dosage requirements may vary based on factors like age, weight, health status, and the specific toxins you're targeting. Consult with a healthcare professional to determine the appropriate dosage for your individual needs.

Manufacturer Reputation: Trustworthy Brands Matter

- **Choose reputable brands:** Opt for supplements and programs from established brands with a proven track record of producing high-quality, safe, and effective products.
- **Look for certifications:** Seek out products that have

been certified by third-party organizations, such as NSF International or USP, which verify the product's quality, purity, and adherence to good manufacturing practices (GMP).

- **Research the company:** Investigate the manufacturer's background, values, and commitment to quality and safety. Look for companies that are transparent about their sourcing, manufacturing processes, and scientific research.

Claims: Separating Hype from Reality

- **Be wary of exaggerated claims:** Be skeptical of products that promise rapid weight loss, "miracle" cures, or unrealistic results. Detoxification is a gradual process that requires a holistic approach.
- **Look for evidence-based claims:** Favor products and programs that base their claims on scientific research and provide references to support their statements.
- **Consult with a healthcare professional:** If you're unsure about a product's claims or safety, seek guidance from a healthcare professional or registered dietitian.

Reading Labels and Identifying Red Flags:

- **Proprietary blends:** Avoid products that list ingredients as part of a proprietary blend, as this obscures the specific amounts of each component.
- **Inadequate information:** Be cautious of labels lacking essential information like serving size, complete ingredient list, manufacturer contact information, or usage instructions.
- **Questionable ingredients:** Steer clear of products containing stimulants, laxatives, diuretics, or other potentially harmful substances.
- **Unsupported claims:** Be skeptical of claims that lack

scientific backing or references to credible research.

By following these guidelines, you can make informed decisions about detox supplements and programs, ensuring that you choose safe, effective, and personalized solutions that support your overall health and well-being. Remember, detoxification is a journey, not a quick fix, and a holistic approach that combines dietary changes, lifestyle modifications, and targeted interventions is key to achieving optimal results.

Researching Brands and Companies

Before investing in a detox supplement or program, it's essential to research the brand and company behind the product. Some steps you can take include:

- Visiting the company's website to learn about their manufacturing processes, quality control measures, and commitment to safety and efficacy.
- Looking for third-party certifications, such as GMP or NSF International, which indicate that the company adheres to strict quality and safety standards.
- Reading customer reviews and testimonials to gauge the experiences and satisfaction of other users, while keeping in mind that individual results may vary.
- Consulting with healthcare professionals or reputable organizations, such as ConsumerLab or the Natural Medicines Comprehensive Database, for unbiased information and ratings on specific products.

Consulting with Healthcare Professionals

Before starting any new detox supplement or program, it's crucial to consult with a qualified healthcare professional, such as a naturopathic doctor, functional medicine practitioner, or registered dietitian. They can help you:

- Assess your individual needs and health status to determine if a specific detox approach is appropriate for you.

- Identify potential interactions between detox supplements and any medications or health conditions you may have.
- Recommend safe and effective dosages and durations for detox supplements based on your unique circumstances.
- Monitor your progress and adjust your detox plan as needed to ensure optimal results and minimize the risk of adverse effects.

By taking a thorough and cautious approach to choosing detox products, you can ensure that you are supporting your body's natural detoxification processes in a safe and effective manner.

CHAPTER 15: BUILDING A SUPPORT SYSTEM FOR YOUR DETOX JOURNEY

Embarking on a detoxification journey can be a transformative experience, but it can also present challenges and obstacles along the way. Building a strong support system is essential for staying motivated, overcoming difficulties, and achieving your detox goals.

Finding a Detoxification Buddy or Community

One of the most effective ways to stay accountable and motivated during your detox journey is to find a like-minded buddy or community to share your experiences with. Some ways to connect with others include:

- Joining a local wellness group or detox program that offers group support and resources.
- Connecting with friends, family members, or colleagues who are also interested in detoxification and healthy living.
- Participating in online forums, social media groups, or webinars focused on detoxification and natural health.
- Attending workshops, retreats, or conferences that provide opportunities to learn from experts and connect with others on a similar path.

Having a support system can help you stay committed to your detox goals, provide encouragement during challenging times, and offer valuable insights and advice based on shared experiences.

Connecting with Healthcare Professionals

Building relationships with qualified healthcare professionals who understand and support your detoxification goals is crucial for ensuring a safe and effective journey. Some key practitioners to consider include:

- **Naturopathic doctors:** These physicians are trained in both conventional medicine and natural therapies, and can provide guidance on detoxification protocols, supplements, and lifestyle modifications.
- **Functional medicine practitioners:** These healthcare providers focus on identifying and addressing the root causes of health issues, and can help develop personalized detox plans based on your unique needs and circumstances.
- **Registered dietitians:** These nutrition experts can provide guidance on detox-friendly diets, nutrient balance, and meal planning to support your body's natural cleansing processes.
- **Holistic therapists:** Practitioners such as acupuncturists, massage therapists, and chiropractors can offer complementary therapies that support detoxification and promote overall well-being.

Establishing open and collaborative relationships with your healthcare team can help ensure that your detox journey is tailored to your individual needs and that you have access to expert guidance and support throughout the process.

Joining Online Forums and Support Groups

In addition to in-person connections, online forums and support groups can be valuable resources for learning, sharing, and finding encouragement during your detox journey. Some benefits of participating in online communities include:

- Access to a wide range of experiences, insights, and perspectives from people at various stages of their detox journeys.
- Ability to ask questions, seek advice, and receive support from others who understand the challenges and triumphs of detoxification.
- Opportunities to learn about new resources, products, and strategies for optimizing your detox results and overall health.
- A sense of connection and belonging, even if you don't have access to in-person support or live in a remote area.

When participating in online forums or support groups, be mindful of the quality and credibility of the information shared, and always consult with your healthcare team before making any significant changes to your detox plan.

Staying Motivated and Overcoming Challenges

Maintaining motivation and navigating challenges is a natural part of any detoxification journey. Some strategies for staying inspired and resilient include:

- Setting clear, achievable goals and celebrating your progress along the way, no matter how small.
- Keeping a journal to track your experiences, insights, and breakthroughs, and to reflect on your growth and achievements.
- Practicing self-care and stress management techniques, such as meditation, deep breathing, or gentle exercise, to support your physical, mental, and emotional well-being.
- Seeking inspiration from books, podcasts, or videos that align with your detox goals and values.
- Maintaining a positive, compassionate mindset and embracing setbacks as opportunities for learning and growth.

Remember that detoxification is a journey, not a destination, and that your experiences and challenges are unique to you. By building a strong support system and staying connected to your intentions and values, you can navigate the ups and downs of your detox journey with greater ease and resilience.

APPENDIX

Resources for Further Information

- Environmental Working Group (EWG): A non-profit organization that provides information on toxins in food, personal care products, and household items, as well as guidance on making safer choices. (https://www.ewg.org/)
- Natural Medicines Comprehensive Database: A reliable source of evidence-based information on natural medicines, including herbs, supplements, and other complementary therapies. (https://naturalmedicines.therapeuticresearch.com/)
- ConsumerLab: An independent organization that tests and reviews dietary supplements and provides unbiased information on their quality, purity, and efficacy. (https://www.consumerlab.com/)
- Institute for Functional Medicine (IFM): A leading organization in the field of functional medicine, offering education, resources, and tools for healthcare practitioners and individuals interested in a systems-based approach to health and wellness. (https://www.ifm.org/)
- National Center for Complementary and Integrative Health (NCCIH): A U.S. government agency that provides reliable, science-based information on complementary and integrative health practices, including detoxification. (https://www.nccih.nih.gov/)

Glossary of Detoxification Terms

- **Antioxidants:** Compounds that help protect cells from damage caused by free radicals and oxidative stress, and support the body's natural detoxification processes.
- **Bioaccumulation:** The gradual accumulation of toxins in the body over time, often due to chronic exposure to low levels of environmental pollutants.
- **Detoxification:** The process by which the body identifies, neutralizes, and eliminates toxins and waste products through various physiological pathways.
- **Endocrine disruptors:** Chemicals that can interfere with the body's hormonal systems, potentially leading to health issues such as reproductive disorders, developmental problems, and certain types of cancer.
- **Free radicals:** Highly reactive molecules that can cause cellular damage and contribute to oxidative stress, inflammation, and chronic disease.
- **Glutathione:** A powerful antioxidant produced by the body that plays a crucial role in detoxification, immune function, and cellular protection.
- **Heavy metals:** Toxic elements such as mercury, lead, arsenic, and cadmium that can accumulate in the body and contribute to various health issues.
- **Leaky gut syndrome:** A condition characterized by increased intestinal permeability, which can allow toxins, bacteria, and partially digested food particles to enter the bloodstream, triggering inflammation and immune responses.
- **Microbiome:** The collection of microorganisms, including bacteria, fungi, and viruses, that inhabit the human body and play crucial roles in digestion, immunity, and overall health.
- **Phytochemicals:** Naturally occurring compounds found in plants that offer various health benefits, including antioxidant, anti-inflammatory, and detoxification support.
- **Xenobiotics:** Foreign substances, such as drugs, pesticides,

and other synthetic chemicals, that can be detrimental to human health when accumulated in the body.

This concludes our comprehensive guide on detox diets for the modern age. By understanding the importance of detoxification, implementing targeted strategies, and building a strong support system, you can embark on a transformative journey towards optimal health and well-being. Remember to always consult with qualified healthcare professionals and trust your body's innate wisdom as you navigate the path of detoxification and self-discovery.

Disclaimer

This book is intended for informational purposes only and should not be construed as professional advice. The information contained herein is not a substitute for professional guidance from qualified individuals in the relevant fields.

You are advised to consult with appropriate professionals, including but not limited to:

- **Healthcare professionals** for any health-related matters.
- **Business professionals** for financial, legal, or business advice.
- **Other relevant experts** in any field related to the topics discussed in this book.

The author and publisher make no warranties or representations, express or implied, with respect to the accuracy, completeness, or timeliness of the information contained in this book. The author and publisher disclaim all liability for any loss or damage resulting from the use or reliance on the information presented in this book.

This book is provided "as is" and without warranty of any kind, express or implied, including but not limited to warranties of merchantability, fitness for a particular purpose, and non-infringement.

It is your responsibility to independently verify any information presented in this book and seek professional advice as needed.

For other books and resources that may interest you, please click here:

https://know.howtobeon.top/gertrudeswanson

www.ingramcontent.com/pod-product-compliance
Lightning Source LLC
Chambersburg PA
CBHW051648250726
48653CB00007B/2555